# Weight Management Strategies

## Maintaining Weight loss and Embracing a healthy Lifestyle

By

## Noah Emberwood

# Table of Contents

# Introduction

## Chapter 1: Understanding Weight Management

Maintaining a healthy weight is not just about aesthetics; it has a crucial role in boosting overall well-being and reducing the risk of chronic diseases. Understanding weight management needs a holistic approach that spans numerous elements, from diet and physical exercise to psychology and genetics. In this chapter, we will study the importance of healthy weight, the factors impacting weight gain and decrease, and the numerous components involved in efficient weight control.

**1.1 The Importance of Healthy Weight:**

Weight control extends beyond social ideas of attractiveness and aesthetics. Achieving and maintaining a healthy weight is vital for boosting quality of life and preventing a multitude of health concerns. Excess weight, particularly obesity, is related with an increased risk of heart disease, type 2 diabetes, some malignancies, and other health difficulties. Conversely, being underweight can also contribute to dietary deficits and reduced immunological function. Recognizing the importance of maintaining a healthy weight motivates individuals to embark on a weight management path that focuses on long-term well-being.

## 1.2 Factors Affecting Weight Gain and Loss:

Weight management is a complicated interplay of numerous elements, and understanding these influences is vital for efficient weight control. Genetics plays a role in defining body size and shape, but it does not control one's fate. Lifestyle factors, such as nutrition and physical activity, substantially effect weight. Hormones, such insulin and leptin, regulate hunger and fat storage, making hormonal balance a key concern in weight management. Additionally, sleep quality, stress levels, and metabolic rate contribute to the delicate equilibrium of weight regulation.

## 1.3 Body Mass Index (BMI) and Its Limitations:

Body Mass Index (BMI) is a regularly used tool to assess if an individual's weight falls within a healthy range. It is computed by dividing a person's weight in kilograms by the square of their height in meters. While BMI provides a basic estimate of body composition, it has limits. It doesn't account for elements such as muscle mass, bone density, and distribution of body fat. As a result, persons with larger muscle mass may be classed as overweight or obese by BMI despite having a good body composition.

## 1.4 Setting Realistic Weight Goals:

Embarking on a weight management journey entails setting reasonable and achievable goals. It is crucial to remember that weight loss and maintenance may not happen immediately. Establishing short-term and long-term objectives helps to sustain motivation and monitor progress effectively. Realistic goals incorporate individual preferences, lifestyle, and medical problems. A gradual and sustainable approach to weight management provides better adherence and long-term success.

## 1.5 The Role of Caloric Balance:

Caloric equilibrium sits at the core of weight management. It refers to the balance between the calories taken through food and beverages and the calories dissipated through physical activity and metabolism. To lose weight, one must generate a caloric deficit, which involves taking fewer calories than the body utilizes. Conversely, to acquire weight, a calorie surplus is necessary. Understanding caloric balance helps individuals to make informed decisions regarding their food and exercise levels, leading to optimal weight control.

## 1.6 Exploring Different Weight Management Approaches:

Numerous weight management treatments and diets exist, each claiming to be the most efficient. It is crucial to approach weight control with a critical and informed perspective. Fad diets that promise rapid solutions generally lack sustainability and may lead to nutritional deficits. Instead, concentrating on balanced and whole-food-based eating habits, such as the Mediterranean or DASH diet, fosters healthy and sustained weight management.

## 1.7 The Connection Between Physical Activity and Weight:

Physical activity has a significant function in weight management. Regular exercise not only burns calories but also raises metabolic rate, improves insulin sensitivity, and sustains lean muscle mass. Combining cardiovascular workouts with strength training activities is an efficient strategy to increase weight loss while retaining muscle mass. Integrating physical exercise into daily life, such as walking or using the stairs, also helps to overall energy expenditure.

## 1.8 Psychological Aspects of Weight Management:

Weight management is not simply about physical aspects; psychology plays a big part as well. Emotional eating, stress, and self-image can influence eating behaviors and weight-related choices. Developing mindfulness around food, understanding emotional triggers, and adopting good coping methods are critical components of successful weight management. Building a healthy relationship with food and body creates a positive mentality and sustainable habits.

**1.9 Seeking Professional Guidance:**

Individuals embarking on a weight management journey can benefit from getting help from healthcare specialists, such as licensed dietitians or nutritionists. These specialists can provide specialized guidance and support tailored to individual requirements and goals. They can assist clients understand their dietary requirements, design proper meal plans, and make sustainable lifestyle adjustments for long-term weight management success.

In conclusion, understanding weight management takes a multidimensional approach that includes numerous aspects impacting weight increase and decrease. It entails setting realistic objectives, understanding the significance of caloric balance, adding physical activity, and treating psychological elements. By taking a complete approach to weight management, individuals can achieve not only a healthy weight but also general well-being and increased quality of life.

# Part I: Nutrition for Weight Management

## Chapter 2: Building a Balanced Plate

Creating a balanced plate is the foundation of a healthy and nutritious diet. A well-balanced meal provides the body with needed nutrition, energy, and satiety while supporting weight management goals. In this chapter, we will cover the fundamentals of making a balanced plate, the value of each food group, and practical strategies for incorporating balanced meals into daily living.

### 2.1 Understanding the Components of a Balanced Plate:

A balanced meal normally consists of three primary components: proteins, carbs, and vegetables (or fruits). Each of these components performs a distinct role in providing critical nutrients and promoting overall health. Proteins are needed for tissue healing, muscle maintenance, and hormone production. Carbohydrates serve as the primary source of energy, supporting brain function and physical activities. Vegetables and fruits are rich in vitamins, minerals, antioxidants, and fiber, which are necessary for appropriate digestion, immunological function, and general well-being.

## 2.2 The Importance of Macronutrients:

Macronutrients, which include proteins, carbs, and fats, are the building blocks of a balanced meal. Understanding their responsibilities and establishing a healthy balance is vital for overall health and weight management. Proteins help to maintain and repair tissues, boost the immune system, and increase satiety. Healthy sources of protein include lean meats, poultry, fish, beans, tofu, and dairy products. Carbohydrates provide the body with easily available energy and should include whole grains, fruits, vegetables, and starchy meals. Healthy fats, found in avocados, nuts, seeds, and olive oil, are needed for hormone balance, nutrition absorption, and cell structure.

## 2.3 The Power of Micronutrients:

Micronutrients, such as vitamins and minerals, are needed for many physiological functions in the body. Incorporating a variety of colored fruits and vegetables into the diet ensures a wide range of micronutrients that support optimal health. Vitamins like A, C, and E work as antioxidants, protecting cells from damage. Minerals including calcium, iron, and potassium are necessary for bone health, oxygen delivery, and neuron function. A balanced plate is rich in micronutrients, improving overall well-being and minimizing the risk of chronic diseases.

## 2.4 Portion Control and Mindful Eating:

Building a balanced plate also entails portion control and careful eating. Being conscious of hunger and fullness cues helps prevent overeating and creates a healthier relationship with food. Paying attention to the quantity of portions and utilizing smaller plates can aid in portion control. Taking time to taste each meal and eating slowly can boost satisfaction and lessen the inclination to overindulge. Mindful eating increases enjoyment and appreciation of the food we consume, encouraging a healthy and balanced approach to eating.

## 2.5 Customizing Meals to Individual Needs:

There is no one-size-fits-all strategy to producing a balanced plate. Individual needs, tastes, and dietary limitations should be considered when designing meals. For example, athletes may require more protein and carbohydrates to sustain their busy lifestyle, while those with specific medical issues may need to avoid certain foods. Understanding one's specific dietary requirements and adjusting meals accordingly ensures that the balanced plate is both enjoyable and supportive of individual health goals.

## 2.6 Incorporating Balanced Snacks:

In addition to balanced meals, having balanced snacks between meals can assist maintain energy levels and reduce overeating during main meals. Balanced snacks contain a combination of macronutrients and micronutrients to give sustained energy and satiety. Nutritious snack options include a handful of almonds with a piece of fruit, Greek yogurt with berries, or carrot sticks with hummus. Snacking carefully and choosing nutrient-dense alternatives adds to a well-rounded diet.

## 2.7 The Role of Hydration:

Hydration is a crucial part of a balanced plate and general wellness. Drinking a proper amount of water throughout the day is crucial for digestion, nutrient absorption, temperature regulation, and maintaining energy levels. Water is the best choice for hydration, however herbal teas and infused water can offer diversity to the fluid intake.

In conclusion, establishing a balanced plate is a cornerstone of a healthy diet and weight management. Understanding the importance of macronutrients and micronutrients, practicing portion control and mindful eating, and adapting meals to individual needs are critical steps towards achieving balanced nutrition. By combining a range of nutrient-dense meals and drinking adequately, individuals can build a sustainable and healthy approach to eating, supporting overall health and well-being.

# Chapter 3: Designing an Effective Meal Plan

Designing an effective meal plan is a strategic strategy to provide balanced nutrition, support weight management goals, and foster good eating habits. In this chapter, we will discuss the basic parts of establishing a personalized meal plan, including assessing caloric needs, setting nutritional goals, and combining a range of foods to support maximum health and well-being.

## 3.1 Assessing Individual Nutritional Needs:

The first stage in establishing a meal plan is to determine individual nutritional needs. Factors such as age, gender, weight, height, activity level, and health issues play a key influence in determining calorie requirements and nutrient consumption. Consulting with a qualified dietitian or nutritionist can give a full review of individual needs and assist adapt the food plan accordingly.

## 3.2 Understanding Macronutrient Distribution:

Determining the distribution of macronutrients (proteins, carbs, and fats) is a critical element of an effective meal plan. The amounts of macronutrients might vary dependent on individual goals, such as weight loss, muscle gain, or general well-being. Striking a balance between these macronutrients provides energy balance, supports physiological functioning, and regulates appetite and fullness.

## 3.3 Emphasizing Whole Foods and Nutrient Density:

Whole foods, rich in critical nutrients and minimally processed, should be the foundation of an effective meal plan. Fruits, vegetables, whole grains, lean proteins, and healthy fats supply a diverse spectrum of vitamins, minerals, antioxidants, and fiber that promote general health. Prioritizing nutrient-dense foods optimizes nutritional intake without unnecessary calories.

## 3.4 Creating Balanced Meals:

A balanced meal consists of a variety of food types to guarantee a well-rounded nutrient intake. A plate should include a dish of lean protein (e.g., poultry, fish, tofu), a portion of complex carbs (e.g., whole grains, legumes), and a generous number of colorful vegetables or fruits. Incorporating healthy fats, such as avocado or olive oil, significantly boosts the nutritional profile of the meal.

## 3.5 Meal Prepping & Planning Ahead:

Meal prepping and planning ahead are helpful techniques to preserve consistency and avoid bad eating choices. Batch cooking and preparing meals in advance can save time and lessen the likelihood of reaching for less nutritious options when in a rush. Creating a weekly meal plan and shopping list streamlines the process and encourages adherence to the targeted nutritional goals.

## 3.6 Mindful Eating and Portion Control:

Mindful eating techniques, such as eating deliberately and appreciating each meal, contribute to better digestion and enhanced satisfaction. Portion control is crucial to prevent overeating and maintain a balanced caloric intake. Using smaller plates and being aware of hunger and fullness cues can help thoughtful and appropriate portion sizes.

## 3.7 Incorporating Cultural and Personal Preferences:

An efficient meal plan should reflect individual cultural and personal dietary preferences. Embracing familiar and tasty foods improves adherence to the plan and enhances satisfaction with meals. Integrating new dishes and cuisines can also offer variety and excitement to the dining experience.

## 3.8 Hydration and Beverage Choices:

Proper hydration is vital to overall health and well-being. Incorporating an adequate intake of water throughout the day is vital. Additionally, being conscious of beverage choices, such as reducing sugary drinks and alcohol, leads to a healthy meal plan.

## 3.9 Adjusting the Meal Plan as Needed:

A meal plan should not be inflexible; it should be adaptive to fit changing demands and circumstances. Life events, exercise levels, and health conditions might change food requirements. Regularly reassessing and changing the meal plan ensures that it remains aligned with individual goals and tastes.

In conclusion, developing an efficient meal plan takes a careful and tailored approach. By assessing individual nutritional needs, emphasizing whole foods, making balanced meals, and practicing mindful eating, individuals can establish healthy eating habits and assist their weight management journey. An adaptive and well-planned meal strategy increases general well-being and leads to a sustainable and joyful relationship with food.

# Chapter 4: Managing Emotional Eating

Emotional eating is a widespread phenomenon when individuals utilize food as a strategy to cope with emotions, stress, or other psychological stimuli rather than eating in reaction to physical hunger. It can lead to unhealthy eating practices and weight management issues. In this chapter, we will explore tactics and approaches to effectively manage emotional eating, build a healthier connection with food, and promote mindful eating habits.

## 4.1 Understanding Emotional Eating:

Emotional eating is utilizing food to calm negative feelings, such as stress, boredom, melancholy, loneliness, or worry. It is generally a response to emotional cues rather than bodily hunger. Recognizing emotional eating patterns is the first step toward building healthier coping methods and stopping the cycle of using food to regulate emotions.

## 4.2 Identifying Emotional Triggers:

Identifying emotional triggers is key in managing emotional eating. Keeping a food journal or an emotional diary can assist track eating patterns and identify situations, feelings, or events that lead to emotional eating episodes. Understanding these triggers allows individuals to build targeted methods to address the fundamental causes of emotional eating.

## 4.3 Developing Alternative Coping Strategies:

Finding alternate coping skills to manage emotions without turning to food is vital for stopping the emotional eating loop. Techniques such as deep breathing, meditation, physical activity, writing, or talking to a friend or therapist can give better outlets for stress and emotions. Engaging in hobbies and activities that bring joy and fulfillment can also serve as useful distractions from emotional eating.

## 4.4 Mindful Eating Practices:

Mindful eating encourages a conscious and present awareness of eating patterns and experiences. Practicing mindfulness during meals requires savoring each bite, eating carefully, and paying attention to hunger and fullness indicators. By being more attentive to the body's demands, individuals can discern between emotional hunger and physical hunger, lessening the possibility of turning to food as a coping mechanism.

## 4.5 Creating a Supportive Food Environment:

Creating a supportive food environment at home and work can assist manage emotional eating. Stocking the pantry and refrigerator with healthful and tasty foods lessens the temptation to indulge in poor choices during stressful periods. Surrounding oneself with positive influences and supportive friends can also develop healthy eating habits and mental well-being.

## 4.6 Managing Stress:

Stress management is a vital element of regulating emotional eating. Implementing stress-reducing activities, such as frequent physical activity, yoga, or mindfulness practices, can lessen the risk of utilizing food to cope with stress. Prioritizing self-care and finding time for relaxation and rejuvenation is vital for emotional well-being.

## 4.7 Seeking Professional Support:

For individuals struggling with emotional eating, obtaining professional support can be beneficial. Registered dietitians, therapists, or counselors can assist address underlying emotional difficulties and provide guidance in creating healthy coping skills. They can also build individualized techniques to regulate emotional eating and encourage long-term behavior change.

## 4.8 Practicing Self-Compassion:

Emotional eating can sometimes lead to emotions of guilt and shame. Practicing self-compassion and self-kindness is vital in breaking free from negative tendencies. Treating oneself with understanding and forgiveness helps establish a healthier relationship with food and encourages beneficial changes in eating behaviors.

## 4.9 Celebrating Progress:

Recognizing and appreciating progress in managing emotional eating is vital for motivation and confidence. Acknowledging modest triumphs and positive adjustments generates a sense of accomplishment and encourages the commitment to sustaining healthier eating habits.

In conclusion, managing emotional eating entails identifying emotional triggers, establishing healthy coping mechanisms, and practicing mindful eating. By creating a supportive food environment, regulating stress, obtaining professional treatment when needed, and embracing self-compassion, individuals can break free from emotional eating patterns and create a healthier and more balanced relationship with food. Developing these methods helps individuals to navigate emotions in a positive and loving way, boosting overall emotional well-being and supporting weight management goals.

# Part II: Exercise and Physical Activity

## Chapter 5: The Role of Exercise in Weight Management

Exercise is a crucial component of a successful weight management journey. It plays a crucial role in burning calories, enhancing metabolic health, and supporting sustained weight loss and maintenance. In this chapter, we will study the role of exercise in weight management, the many types of workouts, and how to incorporate physical activity into daily living.

**5.1 Understanding the Benefits of Exercise for Weight Management:**

Regular exercise gives several benefits for weight management. It helps produce a caloric deficit by burning additional calories, which is vital for weight loss. Exercise also supports the retention of lean muscle mass during weight loss, reducing excessive muscle loss. This is significant since muscle contributes to a higher metabolic rate, helping the body to burn more calories even at rest. Additionally, exercise raises insulin sensitivity, improves cardiovascular health, and promotes general well-being, making it a vital aspect of a comprehensive weight management regimen.

## 5.2 Types of Exercise for Different Goals:

Different types of exercise can be adapted to fit specific weight management goals. Cardiovascular exercises, such as jogging, cycling, swimming, and brisk walking, are helpful for burning calories and boosting cardiovascular fitness. Strength training, encompassing activities like weight lifting and resistance exercises, helps build lean muscle mass and enhances metabolism. Incorporating a combination of aerobic and strength training in a workout regimen ensures a well-rounded approach to weight management.

## 5.3 Creating an Exercise Routine:

Designing an exercise regimen that corresponds with personal interests, physical level, and time limits is vital for long-term adherence. Starting with a realistic workout frequency and gradually increasing intensity can minimize burnout and reduce the chance of injury. Scheduling workouts in advance and making exercise a priority in daily life promotes consistency and ensures a more successful weight management journey.

## 5.4 Incorporating Physical Activity Into Daily Life:

In addition to structured exercise programs, including physical activity into daily living is useful for weight management. Simple actions like climbing the stairs, walking or biking instead of driving short distances, and engaging in home chores can contribute to overall energy expenditure. Being active throughout the day helps enhance non-exercise physical activity, which can have a major impact on overall calorie burn.

## 5.5 Overcoming Barriers to Exercise:

Various impediments can inhibit persons from engaging in regular exercise. Lack of time, motivation, or access to workout facilities are frequent obstacles. Overcoming these limitations demands innovative solutions, such as splitting exercises into shorter periods, discovering engaging kinds of exercise, or researching home training choices. Engaging in physical activities with friends or family can provide social support and enhance motivation.

## 5.6 Listening to the Body and Resting:

Listening to the body's messages and providing it appropriate rest are crucial parts of a balanced exercise plan. Pushing too hard without proper rest can lead to burnout and increased risk of injuries. Rest days are vital for muscle healing and overall physical well-being.

Balancing exercise with rest ensures that physical activity remains sustainable and pleasurable.

## 5.7 Staying Consistent and Setting Goals:

Consistency is crucial to reaching and sustaining weight management goals through exercise. Setting realistic and reasonable exercise objectives, whether it's completing a particular number of exercises per week or increasing the time of physical activity, helps stay motivated and on track. Celebrating accomplishments and achievements along the road creates a good attitude towards exercise and enhances long-term adherence.

## 5.8 Considering Individual Preferences:

Choosing exercise activities that correspond with individual inclinations boosts the likelihood of sticking to an exercise plan. Whether it's dancing, swimming, hiking, or playing a team sport, choosing pleasurable physical activities makes exercise a meaningful and fulfilling element of weight management.

In conclusion, exercise plays a significant role in weight management by enhancing calorie burn, retaining lean muscle mass, and improving overall health. By implementing a combination of cardiovascular and strength training routines, being consistent, and listening to the body's demands, individuals can attain good weight control outcomes. Balancing scheduled exercise with increased everyday physical activity and setting realistic goals promotes a sustainable and enjoyable approach to exercise, supporting overall well-being and weight management success.

# Chapter 6: Combining Cardio and Strength Training

Combining aerobic workouts with strength training is a great technique to obtaining comprehensive fitness and optimizing weight management efforts. This chapter will cover the benefits of integrating both types of workouts, how they compliment each other, and practical ways for implementing them into a well-rounded workout regimen.

6.1 The Synergy of Cardiovascular and Strength Training:

Cardiovascular workouts and strength training each offer specific benefits for the body. Cardio, such as running, cycling, or swimming, boosts heart rate and burns calories, boosting weight loss and cardiovascular health. Strength training, comprising resistance activities like weight lifting, boosts muscular mass, metabolism, and body composition. Combining these two types of exercises provides a potent synergy that enhances general fitness, accelerates calorie burn, and supports sustainable weight management.

## 6.2 Enhancing Caloric Expenditure:

When combined, cardio and strength training enhance caloric expenditure during and after exercise. Cardiovascular workouts burn calories during the activity itself, but strength training induces the "afterburn effect" or excess post-exercise oxygen consumption (EPOC). This means the body continues to burn calories at an elevated rate even after the workout is over. Maximizing caloric expenditure through both types of workouts aids to weight reduction and weight management goals.

## 6.3 Preserving Lean Muscle Mass:

During weight loss, there is a danger of losing both fat and muscle mass. Strength training helps keep lean muscle while reducing excess fat. Maintaining or developing muscle mass is necessary for a greater resting metabolic rate, as muscular tissue requires more energy to sustain than fat tissue. By combining cardio with strength training, individuals can prevent muscle loss and optimize body composition.

## 6.4 Improving Cardiovascular Health:

Cardiovascular workouts are particularly good for increasing heart health, lung capacity, and total cardiovascular fitness. Regular aerobic workouts boost endurance, lower blood pressure, and minimize the risk of heart disease. When linked with strength training, the cardiovascular system becomes more efficient, supporting the body's ability to bear physical demands during exercise and daily activities.

## 6.5 Tailoring Cardio and Strength Workouts:

Tailoring cardio and strength routines to individual interests, fitness levels, and goals is vital for success. Individuals can pick from a wide array of cardio workouts, such as jogging, cycling, dancing, or aerobics. Similarly, strength training can be adapted to use free weights, resistance bands, or bodyweight exercises. By selecting activities that are interesting and demanding, individuals are more likely to adhere to their training schedule.

## 6.6 Frequency and Duration:

Balancing the frequency and duration of aerobic and strength workouts is vital for a well-rounded approach. Aim for at least 150 minutes of moderate-intensity cardio or 75 minutes of vigorous-intensity cardio every week, divided across numerous sessions. Incorporate strength training activities 2-3 times each week, concentrating on different muscle groups. Rest days are vital for muscle healing and overall physical well-being.

## 6.7 Combining Circuit Training:

Circuit training is an efficient approach to integrate both aerobic and strength training into a single session. Circuit training entails executing a sequence of workouts with minimum break in between. It keeps the heart rate raised, offering a cardiovascular challenge, while also including strength workouts that target specific muscle areas. Circuit training optimizes efficiency and time effectiveness in an exercise plan.

## 6.8 Gradual Progression and Periodization:

As with any training plan, moderate progression and periodization are vital for preventing plateaus and reducing the danger of overuse injuries. Gradually increase the intensity, length, or resistance of both cardio and strength training over time. Periodization, or shifting the training focus, helps prevent adaptation and promotes continued growth in fitness and weight control.

## 6.9 Listening to the Body:

Listening to the body's indications and avoiding overtraining are crucial parts of mixing aerobic and strength training. Adequate rest and recovery are necessary for muscle repair and growth. If feeling exhausted or suffering discomfort, consider reducing the intensity or including active rest days into the regimen.

In conclusion, combining cardiovascular workouts and strength training offers a synergistic approach to fitness and weight management. Integrating both types of activities promotes calorie expenditure, preserves lean muscle mass, and improves cardiovascular health. By personalizing workouts to individual interests, gradually progressing, and including circuit training, individuals can construct a well-rounded and effective fitness regimen. Listening to the body and finding delight in workouts develops adherence and adds to long-term success in weight control and overall health.

# Chapter 7: Staying Active Throughout the Day

Incorporating physical activity into daily life extends beyond planned exercise sessions and has a crucial role in promoting general health, weight management, and vitality. This chapter will address the necessity of keeping active throughout the day, practical ways for increasing daily physical activity, and the benefits of incorporating movement into numerous elements of everyday life.

## 7.1 Understanding Non-Exercise Physical Activity:

Non-exercise physical activity, sometimes known as NEPA, refers to the energy used through everyday activities other than formal exercise sessions. These activities include walking, gardening, housework, taking the stairs, and any activity that does not require specific workout time. Accumulating NEPA throughout the day contributes to overall calorie expenditure and aids weight management goals.

## 7.2 Benefits of Non-Exercise Physical Activity:

Engaging in NEPA gives several benefits for physical and mental well-being. It boosts daily energy expenditure, aiding in weight management and reducing weight gain. NEPA enhances cardiovascular health, muscular endurance, and flexibility. Additionally, incorporating activity into daily life might minimize sedentary behavior, which has been connected with bad health effects.

## 7.3 Tips for Increasing Daily Physical Activity:

Increasing everyday physical activity can be accomplished through easy and effective ways. Some recommendations include: - Taking brief walks during work breaks - Opting for active transportation, such as walking or cycling to work - Parking further away from destinations to integrate more walking

- Using stairs instead of elevators or escalators - Doing household chores actively and with purpose - Taking a stroll after meals to improve digestion and increase movement - Engaging in standing or walking meetings wherever possible

**7.4 Setting Activity Reminders:**

Setting activity reminders might be beneficial in building a habit of staying active throughout the day. Using smartphone apps or setting alarms to urge movement breaks at regular intervals can be useful in reducing sedentary behavior. Activity reminders act as incentives to take brief walks, stretch, or undertake easy exercises to break up excessive periods of sitting.

**7.5 Making Movement a Social Activity:**

Incorporating movement into social activities can make remaining active more fun. Engaging in outdoor activities with friends or family, such as hiking, cycling, or playing sports, provides not just physical benefits but also develops social connections. Socializing while being active fosters a healthy attitude towards movement.

**7.6 Embracing Active Leisure:**

During leisure time, engaging active pursuits may be both fun and helpful. Activities like dancing, gardening, playing with pets, or exploring outdoors include movement while offering enjoyment and relaxation. Active leisure pastimes contribute to an active lifestyle without feeling like a chore.

**7.7 Workplace Wellness Initiatives:**

Workplace wellness initiatives can encourage employees in remaining active throughout the day. Employers can encourage NEPA by offering standing desks, creating walking challenges, or providing opportunity for physical exercises during breaks. Workplace support develops a culture of well-being and pushes employees to prioritize mobility in their everyday routines.

**7.8 Family-Friendly Movement:**

Encouraging movement as a family activity offers a favorable environment for remaining active. Family hikes, bike trips, or playing active games together not only boost physical health but also strengthen family bonds. Children learn the value of an active lifestyle through their parents' example.

**7.9 Tracking Progress and Celebrating Achievements:**

Tracking daily physical activity and creating reasonable objectives can help measure progress and keep motivation. Celebrating achievements, whether it's hitting step targets or incorporating more movement into daily life, underscores the significance of keeping active and encourages ongoing effort.

In conclusion, staying active throughout the day by adding non-exercise physical activity gives several benefits for overall health and weight management. Simple tactics like taking short walks, setting activity reminders, and embracing active leisure can greatly affect daily movement. By making movement a social activity and fostering workplace and family support, individuals can develop an active lifestyle that adds to their well-being and long-term weight control success. Tracking progress and celebrating milestones highlight the value of being active and encourage continuous dedication to an active and healthy lifestyle.

# Part III: Lifestyle and Behavioral Changes

## Chapter 8: Setting Realistic Goals

Setting realistic goals is a critical step in any pursuit, including weight control. Realistic goals provide a clear direction, maintain motivation, and develop a sense of achievement. In this chapter, we will explore the necessity of setting realistic objectives, how to establish them effectively, and how they contribute to successful weight management.

**8.1 The Importance of Realistic Goals:**

Realistic goals are vital in weight control to guarantee that the targets are reachable and sustainable. Setting overly ambitious or unrealistic objectives can lead to frustration, disappointment, and a higher risk of giving up. Realistic goals, on the other hand, are practical and feasible, giving a blueprint for continuous progress and long-term achievement.

**8.2 Specific, Measurable, Attainable, Relevant, and Time-Bound (SMART) Goals:**

Adopting the SMART goal-setting framework ensures that goals are well-defined and executable. Each goal should be:

- Specific: Clearly state what you want to achieve and the steps needed to get there.

- Measurable: Set criteria to track progress and determine when the goal is attained.

- Attainable: Ensure that the objective is reasonable and possible based on your existing circumstances and ability.

- Relevant: Align the aim with your weight control objectives and overall well-being.

- Time-Bound: Set a clear deadline for completing the goal, generating a sense of urgency and accountability.

## 8.3 Short-Term and Long-Term Goals:

In weight control, a combination of short-term and long-term goals is important. Short-term goals provide immediate targets and keep you motivated as you attain them. They act as stepping stones towards long-term objectives, which are wider and may require more time and work to attain. Breaking down long-term goals into smaller, doable milestones makes the path more manageable and less stressful.

## 8.4 Tracking Progress:

Regularly assessing progress towards your goals is vital for remaining on course and making modifications as needed. Keep a notebook, use apps, or build spreadsheets to monitor your weight, physical activity, food habits, and other important indicators. Tracking progress provides insights into what is functioning well and indicates areas that may require additional attention.

## 8.5 Celebrating Achievements:

Celebrating victories, no matter how minor, is an essential element of the goal-setting process. Acknowledging and rewarding progress promotes motivation and encourages beneficial behaviour. Celebrations need not be spectacular; they can be as simple as treating yourself to a non-food related reward or taking time to recognize your efforts.

## 8.6 Flexibility and Adaptability:

Life is full of surprises, and situations may change over time. Being flexible and adaptable in your goal-setting method helps you to make required adjustments without losing desire. If you encounter hurdles or endure setbacks, regard them as learning opportunities rather than failures. Modify your goals as needed and continue pushing forward with conviction.

## 8.7 Seeking Professional Guidance:

If you find it tough to set realistic goals or require specialized direction, finding support from a certified dietitian, nutritionist, or fitness professional might be valuable. They can help you develop reasonable objectives, adjust your weight management plan to your unique needs, and provide continuing support and encouragement.

## 8.8 Cultivating Patience and Persistence:

Weight control is a journey that demands patience and persistence. Sustainable growth takes time, and it's crucial to stay committed to your goals even during plateaus or hard moments. Celebrate minor triumphs along the road and remind yourself of the bigger objective — enhancing your health and well-being for the long term.

In conclusion, creating realistic objectives is a vital element of successful weight management. Utilizing the SMART goal-setting framework, establishing short-term and long-term targets, measuring progress, and recognizing achievements are all critical elements in the process. Being flexible and seeking professional help, as well as cultivating patience and persistence, guarantee that you stay on track and reach your weight management goals while nurturing a better and more balanced lifestyle.

# Chapter 9: Sleep and Stress Management

Sleep and stress management are key components of a complete approach to weight management and overall well-being. In this chapter, we will cover the importance of adequate sleep and good stress management, how they impact weight control, and practical techniques to enhance these parts of daily living.

## 9.1 The Impact of Sleep on Weight Management:

Quality sleep plays a key influence in weight management and general health. Insufficient sleep can disturb hormonal balance, leading to increased hunger and cravings for harmful foods. Lack of sleep may also alter the body's capacity to absorb carbohydrates, resulting to abnormalities in blood sugar levels. Adequate and restful sleep supports appropriate metabolism, controls appetite hormones, and contributes to good cognitive function and physical performance.

## 9.2 The Relationship Between Stress and Weight Management:

Stress can be a big hurdle to good weight management. When under stress, the body releases cortisol, a hormone that can stimulate hunger and encourage fat storage, particularly around the abdomen area. Stress eating, or turning to food for comfort during tough times, can also contribute to consuming additional calories and adopting less nutritional food choices. Managing stress correctly is vital for maintaining good eating habits and general well-being.

## 9.3 Strategies for Improving Sleep Quality:

Improving sleep quality is vital for weight management and overall health. Some techniques to promote better sleep include: - Maintaining a consistent sleep schedule by going to bed and waking up at the same time every day, especially on weekends.

- Creating a peaceful bedtime ritual, such as reading, listening to quiet music, or practicing meditation.

- Creating a sleep-conducive environment by keeping the bedroom cold, dark, and quiet.

- Limiting screen time and avoiding stimulating activities close to bedtime.

- Avoiding large meals, caffeine, and alcohol before night, as these can interfere with sleep quality.

## 9.4 Techniques for Effective Stress Management:

Effective stress management can lessen its detrimental impact on weight control and general health. Some stress management approaches include: - Regular physical activity, such as yoga, walking, or meditation, which helps reduce stress hormones and promote relaxation.

- Deep breathing exercises and mindfulness activities to calm the mind and alleviate tension.

- Engaging in hobbies and activities that offer joy and provide an outlet for stress.

- Setting realistic expectations and learning to prioritize chores to reduce feelings of overload.

- Seeking help from friends, family, or professional counselors to talk about stressors and obtain new perspectives.

## 9.5 Creating a Bedtime Routine:

Establishing a consistent bedtime ritual might inform the body that it's time to wind down and prepare for sleep. Activities like reading, having a warm bath, or doing relaxation exercises can enhance relaxation and improve sleep quality.

## 9.6 Incorporating Physical Activity:

Regular physical activity not only improves weight management but also helps reduce stress and enhance sleep quality. Engaging in moderate-intensity exercise, such as walking or yoga, can have favorable benefits on both stress levels and sleep patterns.

## 9.7 Mindfulness and Meditation:

Mindfulness activities and meditation can help individuals manage stress, enhance focus, and encourage better sleep. Practicing mindfulness involves being present in the moment and accepting thoughts and feelings without judgment, which can be particularly useful in reducing stress.

## 9.8 Prioritizing Self-Care:

Prioritizing self-care is vital for both stress management and decent sleep. Taking time to indulge in activities that promote relaxation, joy, and well-being can dramatically improve overall health and weight management efforts.

## 9.9 Seeking Professional Support:

If sleep difficulties or stress become chronic and significantly impair everyday living, receiving support from healthcare professionals, such as sleep specialists or therapists, is suggested. They can provide individualized techniques to address specific sleep or stress-related difficulties.

In conclusion, sleep and stress management are key aspects in weight management and overall health. Improving sleep quality, adopting appropriate stress management practices, and emphasizing self-care contribute to a balanced and successful approach to weight management. By implementing these practices into daily life, individuals can develop a better and more sustainable lifestyle, supporting both physical and emotional well-being.

# Chapter 10: Creating a Supportive Environment

Creating a supportive atmosphere is a critical aspect in achieving successful weight management and fostering a healthy lifestyle. In this chapter, we will discuss the relevance of a supportive environment, how it influences behavior and choices, and practical strategies to build a setting that encourages healthy habits and general well-being.

**10.1 The Role of Environment in Weight Management:**

The place we dwell in substantially influences our behaviour, including eating and physical exercise patterns. A supportive environment can make it simpler to acquire and sustain healthy behaviors, whereas an unsupportive setting might hamper growth. By structuring our environment to correspond with our health and weight management goals, we enhance the likelihood of success and favorable outcomes.

**10.2 Designing a Healthy Food Environment:**

Creating a healthy food environment at home and in the workplace is vital for supporting weight management. Some options include: - Stocking the pantry and refrigerator with nutritious and wholesome foods, such as fruits, vegetables, whole grains, lean meats, and healthy fats.

- Keeping harmful, high-calorie snacks out of sight and replacing them with better ones.

- Preparing healthy meals and snacks in advance to avoid the temptation of ordering takeout or ingesting less nutritious options when time is short.

## 10.3 Encouraging Physical Activity:

A friendly setting should encourage physical exercise and make it accessible. Some ways to do this include: - Designing an exercise environment at home with exercise equipment or workout tools.

- Choosing a workplace that fosters physical exercise, such as allowing standing workstations or providing opportunity for active breaks.

- Encouraging active transportation, such as walking or cycling, by making it a convenient and enjoyable choice.

## 10.4 Social Support and Accountability:

Social support plays a significant role in weight management success. Surrounding oneself with helpful others who share similar health goals can bring encouragement and motivation. Creating or joining support groups, exercise courses, or online communities can offer a sense of accountability and companionship in the road towards improved health.

## 10.5 Minimizing Temptations:

Minimizing temptations in the environment might assist avoid poor dietary choices. For example: - Limiting the presence of sugary snacks, sugary beverages, and high-calorie goodies at home or in the workplace.

 - Avoiding places with considerable food temptations, such as fast-food restaurants or buffet-style settings.

## 10.6 Mindful Eating Practices:

Promoting mindful eating practices within the environment can increase overall well-being. Encourage taking time to savor meals, eating without distractions, and responding to hunger and fullness cues. A mindful eating strategy develops a healthier relationship with food and helps weight management goals.

## 10.7 Creating a Positive Atmosphere:

Fostering a happy atmosphere in the home and workplace can have a big impact on overall well-being.

Encourage positivity, gratitude, and open communication to minimize stress and build a healthy mentality.

## 10.8 Flexibility and Adaptability:

An setting that supports weight management should be flexible and responsive to changing conditions and individual needs. Recognize that life events and schedules may sometimes disturb patterns, and be prepared to change and find balance accordingly.

## 10.9 Celebrating Success and Progress:

Celebrate victories, both big and small, during the weight management journey. Acknowledging achievements encourages beneficial behaviors and boosts motivation to continue making healthy choices.

In conclusion, having a supportive environment is vital for successful weight management and overall well-being. By building a healthy food environment, encouraging physical activity, finding social support, and promoting mindful eating practices, individuals can set themselves up for long-term success. Minimizing temptations, promoting a pleasant attitude, and being flexible and adaptive contribute to a supportive environment that develops healthier behaviors and enhances the overall quality of life.

# Part IV: Dealing with Plateaus and Challenges

## Chapter 11: Overcoming Weight Loss Plateaus

Weight reduction plateaus are regular occurrences along the weight management journey, where progress seems to stall despite persistent efforts. In this chapter, we will investigate the causes of weight loss plateaus, techniques to overcome them, and how to retain motivation during these hard stages.

**11.1 Understanding Weight Loss Plateaus:**

Weight loss plateaus are periods of time when the scale does not reflect any substantial changes while keeping a healthy diet and exercise plan. They might be irritating and demotivating, but they are a natural part of the weight management process. Plateaus typically arise when the body adapts to new habits and changes its metabolism to conserve energy.

**11.2 Analyzing Habits and Patterns:**

When reaching a weight reduction plateau, it is vital to review food and exercise habits. Keep a food journal to document calorie consumption, meal composition, and portion sizes. Review your exercise program and assess whether it needs adjustments to challenge the body in new ways.

## 11.3 Avoiding Monotony in Exercise:

Switching up the exercise program can help break past a plateau. The body adapts to repetitive motions, so increasing variation and trying new exercises can test different muscle groups and raise calorie expenditure.

## 11.4 Adjusting Caloric Intake:

As the body loses weight, its caloric needs may decrease. Reevaluate your caloric intake and alter it to suit your current weight and exercise level. Avoid significantly decreasing calories, as it might lead to vitamin deficits and slow down metabolism.

## 11.5 Incorporating Strength Training:

Incorporating strength training routines might be particularly effective during a weight reduction stall. Building muscle raises the body's metabolic rate, encouraging calorie burn even at rest. Strength training can also assist preserve muscle mass after weight loss.

## 11.6 Being Mindful of Portion Sizes:

Even with healthy meal choices, portion sizes matter. Be conscious of portion sizes to avoid unwittingly overeating, especially when presented with calorie-dense foods.

## 11.7 Ensuring Adequate Hydration:

Proper hydration is vital for general health and weight management. Drinking adequate water can help avoid water retention and promote metabolism.

## 11.8 Managing Stress:

Stress can alter hormone levels and potentially contribute to weight loss plateaus. Engaging in stress-reducing methods, such as meditation, yoga, or spending time in nature, might be useful during plateaus.

## 11.9 Staying Patient and Persistent:

Weight reduction plateaus can be depressing, but it's vital to stay patient and consistent. Remember that weight control is a journey with ups and downs. Stay focused on making healthy choices and trust that growth will restart.

## 11.10 Celebrating Non-Scale Victories:

While the scale may not show instant progress, enjoy non-scale victories, such as greater energy levels, improved fitness, or good changes in body composition. These achievements are equally essential measures of growth.

## 11.11 Seeking Support:

If you feel trapped in a weight reduction plateau, receiving advice from a certified dietitian, nutritionist, or fitness expert can be beneficial. They can provide personalized counsel, support, and inspiration to assist overcome plateaus and sustain growth.

In conclusion, weight loss plateaus are frequent during weight management, but they can be overcome with persistence and alterations to habits and routines. Analyzing routines, modifying calorie intake, including strength training, and controlling stress are excellent techniques to break through plateaus. Celebrating non-scale wins and seeking support during hard times can help sustain motivation and keep you on track towards your weight management objectives. Remember that weight control is a journey, and it's crucial to stay patient and persistent throughout the process.

# Chapter 12: Maintaining Weight Loss

Maintaining weight loss is a key part of good weight management. After accomplishing weight loss goals, it's vital to establish lasting practices to prevent weight rebound. In this chapter, we will discuss techniques to maintain weight loss, build a balanced lifestyle, and support long-term success.

## 12.1 Embracing Sustainable Habits:

Sustainable practices are crucial to maintaining weight loss. Focus on establishing lifestyle adjustments that you can keep in the long run, rather than relying on transitory or restricted techniques. Embrace a balanced diet, frequent physical activity, and a happy mindset as the cornerstone of your healthy lifestyle.

## 12.2 Continuing Regular Physical Activity:

Physical activity should remain a significant element of your daily routine even after reaching weight loss goals. Regular exercise helps preserve muscular mass, boosts metabolism, and contributes to general well-being. Find activities you enjoy to make fitness a good and sustainable part of your life.

## 12.3 Practicing Mindful Eating:

Mindful eating is key for maintaining weight reduction. Continue to pay attention to hunger and fullness cues, relish your meals, and avoid distractions during eating. Be cautious of portion sizes and make informed choices regarding the foods you consume.

## 12.4 Monitoring Weight and Progress:

Regularly monitoring your weight and progress can help you stay accountable and spot any potential weight regain early. However, remember that weight swings are typical and focus on overall trends rather than daily changes.

## 12.5 Setting New Goals:

After accomplishing initial weight loss, try setting new goals to maintain your progress and continue improving your health. These goals can include exercise successes, nutritional challenges, or other wellness-related ambitions.

## 12.6 Prioritizing Sleep and Stress Management:

Quality sleep and proper stress management are vital even after achieving weight loss. Prioritize regular sleep and use stress-reduction practices to improve general well-being and prevent stress-related weight gain.

## 12.7 Cultivating a Supportive Environment:

Maintain a friendly environment that encourages healthy habits and supports your weight management goals. Surround yourself with like-minded persons who have similar health ambitions and provide reciprocal encouragement.

## 12.8 Being Patient with Yourself:

Weight maintenance may come with periodic hurdles or setbacks. Be patient with yourself and accept that growth is not always linear. Remember that maintaining weight loss is a lifelong journey, and it's natural to suffer ups and downs.

## 12.9 Celebrating Non-Scale Victories:

Celebrate non-scale successes to celebrate the beneficial changes in your general well-being. Non-scale successes include greater energy levels, more exercise, better mood, and enhanced body confidence.

## 12.10 Avoiding All-or-Nothing Thinking:

Avoid falling into the trap of all-or-nothing thinking. If you suffer a slip-up or diversion from your plan, realize that it's a part of the process. Avoid feeling guilty and use it as an opportunity to learn and make adjustments moving forward.

## 12.11 Seeking Ongoing Support:

Consider getting continuing support from health experts, support groups, or internet forums. Regular check-ins with a certified dietitian or nutritionist can help you stay accountable and receive individualized guidance.

In conclusion, maintaining weight loss involves a commitment to sustainable habits, ongoing physical exercise, and mindful eating. Prioritizing sleep and stress management, setting new goals, and fostering a supportive atmosphere are key for long-term success. Celebrate non-scale achievements, be patient with yourself, and avoid all-or-nothing thinking to create a balanced and positive approach to weight management. Seeking continuing help ensures you have the resources and encouragement needed to maintain your weight loss and enjoy a healthy lifestyle throughout your life journey.

# Conclusion

## Chapter 13: Embracing a Sustainable Healthy Lifestyle

Embracing a sustainable healthy lifestyle extends beyond weight management and covers total well-being. In this chapter, we will discuss the aspects of a sustained healthy lifestyle, the benefits it delivers, and practical techniques to integrate these habits into daily life.

**13.1 Defining a Sustainable Healthy Lifestyle:**

A sustainable healthy lifestyle requires adopting practices that support physical, mental, and emotional well-being in the long run. It promotes balanced eating, frequent physical activity, enough rest, and good stress management. This lifestyle is not centered on short-term diets or drastic methods but focuses on nourishing the body and mind regularly.

**13.2 Balanced Nutrition:**

Eating a balanced and diverse diet is a cornerstone of a sustainable healthy lifestyle. Emphasize entire, nutrient-dense foods such as fruits, vegetables, whole grains, lean meats, and healthy fats. Be cautious of portion sizes, stay hydrated, and limit processed meals, sugary beverages, and excessive salt and added sugars.

## 13.3 Regular Physical Activity:

Incorporate frequent physical activity into your everyday routine. Choose activities you enjoy, whether it's walking, cycling, dancing, or swimming. Aim for at least 150 minutes of moderate-intensity aerobic activity or 75 minutes of vigorous-intensity aerobic activity per week, along with muscle-strengthening activities at least two days a week.

## 13.4 Adequate Rest and Sleep:

Prioritize obtaining enough rest and quality sleep each night. Sleep is vital for physical and mental healing. Aim for 7-9 hours of sleep for most adults, and create a consistent sleep pattern to ensure a healthy sleep-wake cycle.

## 13.5 Effective Stress Management:

Manage stress using numerous strategies such as mindfulness, meditation, yoga, deep breathing, or spending time in nature. Find things that help you relax and unwind, and make stress reduction a regular part of your routine.

## 13.6 Nurturing Relationships:

Cultivate deep ties with friends, family, and a supportive community. Social support is vital for emotional well-being and can favorably benefit physical health.

### 13.7 Enjoyable Physical Activities:

Choose physical activities that provide joy and fulfillment. When you enjoy what you do, it becomes simpler to maintain a regular workout regimen and embrace an active lifestyle.

### 13.8 Being Mindful of Screen Time:

Limit excessive screen time and digital gadget use. Spend more time engaged in face-to-face contacts, outdoor activities, or hobbies that do not involve screens.

### 13.9 Prioritizing Mental Health:

Pay attention to your mental health and seek professional treatment if needed. Regularly exercise self-care, engage in activities that encourage relaxation, and create a happy outlook.

### 13.10 Avoiding Extreme Diets or Restrictive Practices:

Avoid falling into the trap of excessive diets or restrictive behaviors. Embrace a balanced approach to diet and focus on nourishing your body with a variety of healthful meals.

### 13.11 Celebrating Progress:

Celebrate your accomplishments and victories, no matter how minor. Recognize the beneficial changes in your physical health, mental well-being, and entire lifestyle.

## 13.12 Setting Realistic Goals:

Set reasonable and achievable goals that correspond with your values and desires. Break down long-term objectives into smaller, doable tasks to stay motivated and keep concentration.

In conclusion, choosing a sustained healthy lifestyle is a holistic approach to well-being that supports physical health, mental clarity, and general enjoyment. By fueling the body with appropriate nutrition, engaging in regular physical activity, managing stress properly, and prioritizing rest and mental health, you may develop a lifestyle that promotes vitality and fulfillment. Avoid extremes, praise progress, and set realistic goals to guarantee a sustainable and fulfilling journey towards long-term health and happiness.

www.ingramcontent.com/pod-product-compliance
Lightning Source LLC
Chambersburg PA
CBHW071000250726
48663CB00002B/308